100 Plus Essential Oil Healing Recipes

Over 130 Aromatherapy Solutions For Everyday Ailments, Emotional Health And General Well Being

Sandy Comfort

with

Dr. Trey Colton

Disclaimer

The information in this book is solely for informational purposes, not as a medical instruction to replace the advice of your physician or as a replacement for any treatment prescribed by your physician. The author and publisher do not take responsibility for any possible consequences from any treatment, procedure, exercise, dietary modification, action or application of medication which results from reading or following the information contained in this book.

If you are ill or suspect that you have a medical problem, we strongly encourage you to consult your medical, health, or other competent professional before adopting any of the suggestions in this book or drawing inferences from it.

This book and the author's opinions are solely for informational and educational purposes. The author specifically disclaims all responsibility for any liability, loss, or risk, personal or otherwise which is incurred as a consequence, directly or indirectly, of the use and application of any of the contents of this book.

DEDICATION

To Momma, thank you for believing in me.

TABLE OF CONTENTS

INTRODUCTION

Essential oils aren't really oils as they do not contain fatty lipids or acids usually found in animal and vegetable oils. They are in fact, highly concentrated volatile oils extracted from aromatic plants and other sources such as barks, roots, flowers and leaves. They are beautifully and uniquely fragrant and give plants their distinctive smells.

The fragrant residue of a peeled and squeezed orange, for instance is full of essential oil. Additionally, they vary in colors, evaporate easily into the air, absorb effortlessly into the skin when applied and never go rancid.

Healing Effects of Essential Oils

Essential oils have been used for thousands of years to heal and purify the body of ailments and diseases. Its increase in popularity in this present age may not be unconnected with the accessibility of information on the internet.

Additionally, a lot of people are now looking into natural and safe means of maintaining their health and obtaining relief from the very stressful lifestyle that they lead.

Essential oils are an amazing alternative medical treatment. However, they are complimentary and must never be regarded as a substitute to professional medical care.

Aromatherapy alone (the use of essential oils for treatments) cannot cure a major illness or permanently cure your stress. What they do is to help in alleviating the symptoms of a physical condition and to temporarily eliminate stress or other psychological factors.

Not everyone responds to essential oil treatment in the same way. This is because essential oils comprise different characteristics so they should be handled differently. 'Stronger or hotter' oils for instance can cause skin irritation for many people. An essential oil that doesn't irritate you can still irritate someone else.

Also, if you are allergic to a specific plant, there is a tendency for you to also be allergic to the essential oil where it is extracted from. It is advisable to do a skin test to verify its safeness on your skin.

How to Perform a Skin Patch Test

• Combine 1 drop of essential oil and half a teaspoon of carrier oil (olive or jojoba oil will do). Place 1-2 drops of this combination on the inside of your elbow, wrist or underside of the forearm.

• You may apply a bandage to avoid getting the area wet.

• If you feel any irritation, itching or notice some redness, take away the bandage immediately and wash the area carefully.

• If no irritation happens after a few hours, you can go ahead and use the essential oil in diluted form as it is safe on your skin.

Making& Buying Essential Oils

Essential oils are extracted from plants via distillation and cold pressing (expression). Distillation is the most favorable process of essential oil extraction. It involves heating the plant material by passing steam through it or placing it in water which is then heated.

The heat and steam combination slowly beaks down the plant material and the essential oil is thus released. The essential oil components and steam pass through a pipe to a cooling tank where they go back to liquid form and are collected in a container. The essential oil is then separated from the water and stored.

Expression or cold pressing is used to extract oils that are taken from the rinds of fruits like lime, grapefruit, orange, tangerine and lemon. This method is "cold' because it does not require steam or heat of any kind. Instead, mechanical pressure is literally used to squeeze out the oil from the plant material.

The quality of essential oils matter a lot. You need to buy from trusted and reputable source to enjoy effective results. Be wary of mislabeled products. Just because a labeled bottle indicates quality doesn't necessarily mean the content can be trusted.

To test the purity of an essential oil, pour one drop on a clean piece of construction paper. Pure essential oil will evaporate quickly leaving no trace. The presence of a noticeable ring indicates that the oil is diluted.

Diluting Essential Oils With Carrier Oils

Due to essential oils' high concentrative nature, they must be diluted before applying to skin. This can be done effectively with carrier oils.

Carrier oils are pressed from the fatty portions of plants such as the seeds and nuts. As a result, most of them have minimal aroma and minimal color. Some of them also last for a short while as they become rancid after a while.

Carrier oils also act as a lubricating agent during massage of larger areas and muscles. They aid absorption as well. Unlike essential oils that evaporate easily when diluted, carrier oils do not.

Ideal carrier oils for essential oils include olive oil, jojoba, sweet almond oil, pomegranate seed oil, pecan oil, evening primrose oil, hemp seed oil, sesame oil, avocado oil, rose hip oil, sunflower oil and many more.

In order to retain the freshness of your carrier oils, keep them from direct light and heat. Make small batches of blends that can be used within a short time. Jojoba oil is very helpful in extending the shelf life of your blend. Essential and carrier oils can also be refrigerated to extend their shelf life.

A 2% dilution is ideal for most aromatherapy applications. Going beyond this measurement may lead to adverse effect. For children and the elderly and individuals with health issues, just 1% dilution of carrier oil is sufficient.

Lavender or melaleuca oils are very mild and can be used undiluted on skin eruptions and burns. Also, the skin of the foot is so thick it is unaffected by undiluted essential oils when applied in that area. However, this does not mean that the essential oil component did not penetrate into the body.

Guidelines For Essential Oils Usage

Essential oils are not supposed to be applied directly on the skin unless appropriately diluted. This is because the potency of these oils can cause an allergic reaction on people with very sensitive skin. Here are some of the most common ways to use essential oils:

Inhalation

Inhalation method is highly effective for emotional and respiratory issues. It could be direct and indirect. Direct inhalation is physically and psychologically beneficial.

The aroma stimulates the brain to generate a reaction and when it is inhaled straight into the lungs, the natural constituents can provide therapeutic benefit. However, if you are unsure about your level of sensitivity or reaction to a particular use, do a test with only one drop.

Inhalers: has the advantage of mobility and durability. They are easy to purchase, empty inhalers can also be used as the oil drips easily from the wick.

Tissue cup: Place a few tissue or toilet paper inside a small plastic cup with a lid. Drop 5 drops of oil into it. Open the cup occasionally, hold to the nose and breathe deeply. It can last for about 2 weeks. It is highly stimulating and helpful for staying alert in long meetings and when driving.

Cup and Inhale: helps in stimulating the olfactory cells. The cup and inhale method entails placing a few drops of oil on the palm, cupping the hands over the nose and taking a deep breath. The residue on the hands after an external application can also be used.

Make a spritz: combine 5 –10 drops of oil and half a cup of water. Put the mixture into a spray bottle. Shake well before each use.

Make a steam tent: put some drops of oil into a hot bowl of water. Place a towel over the head, allow it drape around the bowl and then breathe in the vapors. This works really well for colds and sinus problems.

Shirt Tent: Apply the oils to the neck and chest and needed. Put on a T-shirt and while in a relaxed position, pull the neck of the shirt up over the nose and then breathe deeply.

<u>Indirect Inhalation – diffusers</u>

Help to release oils into the air. The body easily absorbs the minute ion particles. They have been proven to improve mental clarity and calm emotions.

Topical Application

<u>Direct</u> - Burns, rashes, cuts, bruise fungal, scrapes bumps, infections and bites are some examples of situations where direct topical application is most effective for pain relief and protection from infection.

Topical administration is also perfect on areas of pain and inflammation such as gout, joint pains, arthritics and muscle aches. Same goes for children who suffer from stomach upset. During application however, caution must be observed to avoid contact of undiluted essential oils with the eyes or mucus membranes.

<u>Compresses</u>: Compresses are helpful after an oil massage. Few drops of essential oil are added to a bowl of hot or cold water. A clean, sterile cotton cloth is dipped into the water and rung out. The cloth is then placed on the affected area until the cloth matches the body temperature. In some cases, oils are used with carrier oil.

<u>Massage</u>: Aromatherapy massage can be administered by massage therapists.

<u>Baths and soakings</u> are another way essential oils can be topically applied. Examples of these are saunas, Jacuzzis, baths and showers.

A full bath aids relaxation: Place oils in water; agitate the water from time to time to eliminate concentration of oils in a particular area and immerse inside it.

Foot bath: There are different types of oils and combination for a range of foot ailments. A few drops released into a bowl of warm water that can contain both feet. Mix well and soak as long as comfortable.

Hand soak: Get a smaller container to fit the hands. Reduce the number of drops of oil to mix well with warm water and soak hands for as long as the solution is comfortable.

Ingestion

While essential oils are used in the food and flavoring industry, internal intake of essential oils should be done with professional advice.

Tea - this is the most common method for ingesting essential oils. 1-2 drops of oil is added to a half cup of warm water and sipped or drunk as needed. Water mustn't be too warm otherwise it will dissipate quickly and the potency will be lost.

Water - Oils are usually added to cold water and ingested e.g. using lemon oil due to its cleansing effect.

Capsules – oils can also be added in a capsule and taken orally like traditional medications. Carrier oil may also be added to the capsule as a buffer to the essential oil.

Swishing - a method of adding 2- 6 drops of oils to a teaspoon of water, swishing in the mouth for 40-60 seconds and swallowing.

Insect Repellent

Many essential oils such as peppermint, lavender and citronella act as a natural repellent against insects. To repel insects, sprinkle some drops of essential oil onto tissues or cotton balls and place them near your doors and windows.

Make sure you go through the safety information on the oils you intend to use because some oils may be unsuitable for usage around pets. Also, do not apply the oil directly on fragile surfaces.

Basic Precautions For Essential Oils Usage

- Be careful with sensitive parts of the body like the eyes and ears. On no account should you apply essential oils directly to the ear canal or the eyes. Wash your hand thoroughly after application in order to avoid actions like rubbing the eyes, touching the interior of the nose or handling contact lenses.

- Pregnancy. Although studies have shown that essential oils that are applied topically and after the first trimester cannot harm a developing fetus, it is still advisable to consult a seasoned aromatherapist before usage.

- Some essential oils, mostly citrus oils react to radiant energy, light or other sources of UV rays. Once applied, a rash on the skin or a dark pigmentation shows up within hours or days. It is best to wait for about 6 hours after using any of these photosensitizing oils before exposing the skin to sunlight.

- Be careful with babies and individuals with sensitive skin. Some people naturally have sensitive skin so use common sense. Extra caution should be taken when treating babies, small children, and the elderly. This is because they have very sensitive skin that is prone to burning, irritation or stinging sensations. Protect the skin against irritation by using an effective base or carrier oil.

- Keep Out of Reach of Children. Just as you would for medicine, treat essential oils the same way. Essential oils wrongly ingested are harmful and painful as well if accidentally used in the eyes.

- Most essential oils are flammable so keep them from open flame or spark.

- Also, exercise caution with companies that state their product is "Made With Natural Ingredients" or "Made With Essential Oils". Claims like this do not explicitly state that the product is only made with the specified ingredient. It is possible for such products to contain a tiny amount of essential oil just so that they can make the "Made with Essential Oils" claim.

- The lesser the better. Always remember that these oils are highly concentrated so be sure to follow the exact usage. If one drop can deliver the expected results, do not use two.

Blending Essential Oils

Several essential oils can easily be combined to create a blend that can heal, relax and beautify you. This powerful combination is called a synergy blend. Synergy blend oils are a mix of different oils with harmonizing properties. Utilize these oil blends for your medicinal, aromatherapy and cosmetic purposes.

ESSENTIAL OIL RECIPES FOR DIGESTIVE ISSUES

Acid Reflux/Heartburn/Gerd Abdominal Rub

Eucalyptus essential oil - 2 drops

Peppermint essential oil - 1 drop

Fennel essential oil - 2 drops

Grapeseed oil 1 teaspoon (5ml)

Usage:

1. Mix the essential oils with the carrier oil.

2. Rub on the upper abdominal area whenever you have burning pain in your chest.

Acid Reflux/Heartburn/Gerd Drink

Lemon essential oil - 1 drop

Peppermint essential oil - 1 drop

12-16 oz. of drinking water

Usage

1. Add the oil to your water and drink throughout the day.

2. For an intense episode, add 3 drops of Lemon essential oil to a small glass of warm water and drink.

Diarrhea Relief Massage Oil

Lavender essential oil - 2 drops

Peppermint essential oil - 2 drops

Chamomile essential oil - 2 drops

Geranium essential oil - 2 drops

Eucalyptus essential oil - 2 drops

Vegetable carrier oil - 10 ml

Usage:

1. Combine the ingredients in a dark bottle.

2. Rub over abdominal area twice a day.

Diarrhea Capsule Blend

Oregano essential oil - 2 drops

Mountain savory essential oil - 3 drops

Lemon essential oil - 4 drops

Usage:

1. Add 2-3 drops of this blend to 3 drops of vegetable oil in a 00 size capsule and swallow, twice daily.

Diverticulitis Relief Blend

Individuals above the age of forty can develop diverticulitis when there is continuous pressure against weakened tissue. Drinking Aloe Vera juice 2 or 3 times a day can promote healing.

Rosemary essential oil - 2 drops

Peppermint essential oil - 1 drop

Clove essential oil - 1 drop

Chamomile essential oil - 1 drop

Vegetable carrier oil - 1 teaspoon (5ml)

Usage:

1. Blend essential and carrier oils together.

2. Use as massage oil to relieve the discomfort of the ailment.

Indigestion Digestive Stimulant
Roman Chamomile essential oil - 3 drops

Ginger essential oil - 3 drops

Bergamot essential oil - 5 drops

Grapeseed oil - 1 ounce

Usage:

1. Blend the oils in a bottle then use to massage the stomach and the intestinal area rubbing in a clockwise motion.

2. Alternatively, add 1 drop of Lemon or Fennel essential oil to a cup of Chamomile tea and drink.

Motion Sickness Relief
Motion sickness can be relieved and also prevented by the following blend.

Peppermint essential oil - 10 drops

Ginger essential oil - 10 drops

Roman Chamomile essential oil - 10 drops

Usage:

1. Blend all the essential oils in a dark bottle.

2. Put a few drops on a tissue and breathe in. You can also make use of a personal inhaler.

3. Inhale about 30 to 60 minutes before a journey and every 15 to 30 minutes while traveling.

Nausea Instant Remedy
Try this blend whenever you feel queasy.

Lavender essential oil - 1 drop

Peppermint essential oil - 1 drop

Basil essential oil - 1 drop

Carrier oil - 2 teaspoons (10ml)

Usage:

1. Mix the oils with the carrier oil.

2. Massage gently over your abdomen.

3. Before washing your hands, cup your hands over your mouth and nose and inhale slowly a few times.

Abdominal Pain & Cramps Remedy
This blend is effective for abdominal pain that is caused by eating too fast, inflammation of bladder and other digestive problems. Seek medical advice if the pain persists or if there is fever, vomiting, diarrhea or headache.

Calendula essential oil - 1 drop

Clove oil essential oil - 1 drop

Peppermint essential oil - 1 drop

Carrier oil - 1 teaspoon (5 ml)

Usage:

1. Mix together then massage gently on the stomach area using a clockwise motion.

2. Place a warm washcloth on the massaged area for a few minutes to help intensify the effect of the oil blend.

Flatulence (Gas) Relief Capsule

Ginger essential oil

Lavender essential oil

Carrier oil

Usage:

1. Add 1-2 drops of either of these essential oils to 3-4 drops of vegetable oil in an empty size 00, capsule. Take the capsule 15-30 minutes before eating foods that can cause flatulence.

Flatulence (Gas) Massage Blend

This massage blend is recommended when flatulence is accompanied by pain and discomfort.

Peppermint essential oil ¬- 2 drops

Rosemary essential oil - 3 drops

Clove essential oil - 1 drop

Chamomile essential oil - 1 drop

Olive oil - 1 teaspoon (5ml)

Usage:

1. Rub the blend over your abdominal area two times daily.

Bloating Remedy

Lemongrass or Cypress essential oil - 2 drops

Lemon or Grapefruit essential oil - 4 drops

Grapeseed oil - 1 tablespoon

Usage:

1. Blend oils together properly.

2. Massage the swollen area with upward motions, 2 to 3 times daily.

3. Additionally, drink a glass of water to which 1-2 drops of Lemon essential oil has been added 3 times daily.

Constipation Relief Recipe

You are constipated when bowel movements are fewer than 3 to 4 in a week and you should implement this rectifying procedure.

Peppermint essential oil - 5 drops

Lemon essential oil - 10 drops

Rosemary essential oil - 15 drops

Jojoba oil - 30 ml

Usage:

1. Blend oils together then massage in a clockwise motion over the abdominal area three times a day.

ESSENTIAL OILS FOR RESPIRATORY PROBLEMS

Bronchitis Relief

Bronchitis occurs when the passage ways in the lungs becomes congested and inflamed, causing breathing difficulty.

Sunflower oil- 1 ounce

Eucalyptus essential oil - 12 drops

Peppermint essential oil - 5 drops

Thyme essential oil - 5 drops

Usage:

1. Combine ingredients together

2. Rub gently on your throat and chest several times a day.

Bronchitis Relief For Children

Eucalyptus Radiata essential oil - 10 drops

Myrtle essential oil - 25 drops

Thyme linalool essential oil - 10 drops

Niaouli essential oil - 10 drops

Usage

1. Mix ingredients together.

2. Put 10 drops in a bowl of very hot water and allow the steam to fill the air. Inhaling this steam kills off the germs in the bronchial tubes, trachea and naval cavities.

3. Alternatively, place some drops on a tissue and inhale.

Cold Sores & Fever Blisters Recipe
This blend will enhance healing and reduce the intensity of breakouts.

Roman Chamomile essential oil - 2 drops

Eucalyptus essential oil - 2 drops

Melissa essential oil - 2 drops

Sweet Almond oil - 5 ml

Usage:

1. Mix the ingredients properly.

2. Use a cotton-tip applicator to dab on the blister.

Feet Therapy For Cold & Chilly Feelings
Geranium essential oil - 6 drops

Lemon essential oil - 10 drops

Rosemary essential oil - 4 drops

Usage:

1. Blend together in an amber bottle.

2. Add 3-4 drops to a large basin of hot water. (The water mustn't be too hot)

3. Do not soak feet for more than 30 minutes.

4. Once done, dry your feet well, apply a little lotion.

5. Put on your socks, shoes or slipper.

Essential Oil Therapy For Sinusitis

Sinusitis is a very painful condition that is brought about by various causes such as allergies, colds and the flu. When this happens, the protective mucous membranes that is in your sinus cavities become compromised by germs or other irritants, leading to inflammation and infection.

Steaming water -1 quart

Tea tree essential oil - 2 drops

Eucalyptus essential oil - 2 drops

Thyme essential oil - 1 drop

Ginger essential oil - 1 drop

Usage:

1. Add the essential oils into a 2 quart glass bowl of hot water. (Water mustn't be necessarily steaming).

2. Hold head over the bowl while draping a towel over head and bowl.

3. Breathe for 5 to10 minutes. Repeat this up to 6 times every day.

Nasal Inhaler For Chest Congestion

Eucalyptus essential oil - 5 drops

Coarse salt - 1/4 teaspoon

Usage:

1. Place salt in a small vial with a tight lid. Add essential oil. (The salt absorbs the oil and prevents it from spilling when carried).

2. Open the vial and deeply inhale when needed.

3. Sniff as needed all through the day.

Vapor Rub For Chest Congestion
Eucalyptus essential oil -12 drops

Peppermint essential oil - 5 drops

Thyme essential oil - 5 drops

Olive oil - 1 ounce

Usage:

1. Combine all ingredients in a glass bottle.

2. Shake thoroughly to mix evenly.

3. Massage into chest and throat very gently.

4. Use one to five times daily and just before bed.

Therapy For Wet Throat Cough
Coughs have distinctive characteristics that can be recognized as either good or bad. The originating cause of a "bad" cough may be bacterial, viral or symptomatic of another issue entirely.

Peppermint essential oil - 2 drops

Rosemary essential oil - 2 drops

Lime essential oil - 2 drops

Therapy For Deep Painful Chest Cough
Rosemary essential oil - 2 drops

Eucalyptus essential oil - 2 drops

Frankincense essential oil - 2 drops

Therapy For Dry Hacking Cough
Eucalyptus essential oil - 2 drops

Rosemary essential oil - 2 drops

Lemon essential oil- 2 drops

Usage For All Three:

1. Layer the oils on chest and rub in lightly.

2. While the oils sits on the skin, cup and inhale deeply from your hands for some minutes.

3. Next, pull the neck of your shirt over your nose and mouth. Breathe in deeply for some minutes until the aroma starts to dissipate. (Take breaks and then resume if you feel you aren't getting sufficient oxygen).

4. The oils will penetrate into the lungs and a cooling sensation will be felt.

5. Do this several times on a daily basis.

Tea Remedy For Cough
Clove and lemon essential oil –1 drop each

Water – 8oz

Honey 1-2 drops (to keep water and essential oils from separating).

Extra virgin coconut oil carrier (1 tablespoon, optional)

Usage:

1. Boil water. Add honey and oils to the boiled water. Blend for 60 seconds in a blender at high speed.

2. Keep a toweled head over the steaming cup to enjoy the therapeutic steam.

3. Enjoy the great taste as its travels quickly along the esophagus into the body's organs and inner tissues.

EO Gargle Method For Cough
Eucalyptus, Lemon or Peppermint essential oil - 1- 2 drops

Usage:

1. Put oil(s) in a mouthful (an ounce) of water.

2. Swallow after gargling.

Breathing Rub for Asthma
Common causes of asthma include stress, allergic reactions to food and airborne allergens. The wheezing characterized of asthma is the result of pushing air through swollen and narrowed bronchial passages. The best time to treat asthma is in-between attacks. Do a sniff test first to ensure there is no adverse reaction.

Jojoba oil - 1 oz

Pine needle essential oil - 3 drops

Eucalyptus essential oil - 3 drops

Tea Tree essential oil - 3 drops

Frankincense essential oil - 2 drops

Thyme essential oil - 2 drops

Myrrh essential oil - 2 drops

Usage:

1. Blend all the oils in a clean PET plastic bottle.

2. Rub on the chest and mid back as often as needed.

Essential Oil Steam for Asthma

Eucalyptus essential oil - 1/4 teaspoon

Water - 3 cups

Usage:

1. Boil water and add essential oils. Drape a towel over the back of the head. Place face over steam and breathe in the steam. Take breaks as needed.

2. Do 3 to 4 rounds of steam inhalation several times every day.

Hay Fever And Other Seasonal Allergies

Eucalyptus essential oil - 4 drops

Chamomile essential oil - 4 drops

Anise essential oil - 3 drops

Lemon essential oil - 3 drops

Petitgrain essential oil - 1 drops

Carrier oil - 5 ml

Usage:

1. Blend the oils properly in a dark bottle.

2. Use 15-20 drops in a bath.

ESSENTIAL OILS FOR ACHES & PAINS AROUND THE BODY

Cotton Ball Remedy For Earache

An earache is usually pain in the middle or inner ear. In infants and small children, it is generally the result of irritations brought about by cleaning with a cotton swab or reactions to cleaning products. The trapped fluid puts pressure on the eardrum, causing ache.

Basil essential oil - 3 drops

1/2 of a cotton ball

Grapefruit essential oil - 2 to 3 drops

Usage:

1. Put the basil on a cotton ball and push it into the ear very lightly. (Do not place the oils directly into the ear as vapor from the cotton ball will get to the infected area).

2. Leave it overnight.

3. For additional relief, rub grapefruit oil behind and around the external part of the ear.

4. Place a warm cloth over the ear, while lying down.

Essential Oil Swab Method

Melrose, lavender or tea-tree essential oil: 2-3 drops

Water

Usage:

1. Dilute essential oil with warm water.

2. Swab area around the ear opening, the ear lobe and the exterior part.

Remedy For Mild Tension Headache
A headache is a continuous pain in any region of the head. The brain has pain-sensitive structures and disturbances of these structures causes pain.

Peppermint essential oil – 2-3 drops

Usage:

Rub on the forehead, temples and back of neck.

Remedy For Severe Headache
1. Apply remedy for mild tension headache.

2. Compress the aforementioned areas with a clean, damp towel and rest for a few minutes.

3. Repeat as often as needed. A few drops may be added to the towel to speed up the help.

4. Keep oils away from eyes.

Migraine Headache Hand Soak
Lavender essential oil - 5 drops

Ginger essential oil - 5 drops

Hot water - 1 quart (about 110°F)

Usage:

1. Add the essential oils to the hot water.

2. Soak hands for about 3 minutes.

3. This therapy may be done repeatedly.

Eyelid Swelling (Sty) Remedy
Lavender or chamomile essential oil

Usage:

Dab with cotton wool 2-3 times daily

EO Topical Remedy For Back Pain
Back pain is a common term that covers a wide range of situations primarily around the spinal column.

Birch, deep blue or wintergreen essential oil – 2- 3 drops

Usage:

Apply topically to the area of pain as often as needed.

Remedy For Back Pain Inflammation Reduction
Black Pepper, basil, wintergreen, bergamot or Rosemary essential oil - 2 to 3drops

Usage:

Apply to spinal area topically.

Oils To Increase Circulation In The Back
Geranium, Citrus Bliss, Eucalyptus, Peppermint, Cypress or Lemon essential oil -2 to3 drops

Usage:

Apply topically to spinal area 2 to 3 times per day

Essential Oils To Eliminate Spasms And Relax Muscles

Chamomile, Marjoram, AromaTouch, Lime or Roman essential oil – 2to3 drops

Usage:

Apply topically to the area where the spasm occurs.

Oils To Heal And Regenerate Tissue

Frankincense, Helichrysum or Sandalwood essential oil: 1 -2 drops

Usage:

1. Apply twice or thrice daily and topically to the spinal area.

2. Have a hot compress

EO For Neck Pain Relief

Neck pain usually affects your range of motion. Reduce the spasm and pain in your neck muscles through essential oil application.

Rosemary, peppermint, lavender or juniper essential oil - 5 drops

Usage:

1. Blend the oils in the palm of the hands.

2. Massage mixture into stiff or sore neck.

3. Wrap neck in a scarf for some hours.

Essential Oil Solution For Nose Bleeds

This condition is very common with children. Helichrysum essential oil does not interfere with blood thinning medication.

Helichrysum essential oil- 2- 3 drops

Usage:

1. Apply oil to bleeding nostrils. Apply externally or internally using tissue saturated with helichrysum. The bleeding stops faster with internal application.

Anal Fissures Treatment

These are inflamed tears around the anus caused by straining (usually caused by constipation), excessive rubbing and use of rough toilet paper.

Lavender essential oil - 5 drop

Lemon essential oil - 1 drop

Usage:

1. Add the oils to a bowl of warm water and bathe the area twice daily.

Edema (Swollen Legs, Feet, Ankles, Arms)

This condition occurs as a result of excess fluid in the body tissues at the affected areas. The following blend will strengthen the capillary walls and enhance the drainage of blood.

Cypress essential oil - 3 drops

Lemon essential oil - 5 drops

Grape- seed oil - 1 tablespoon

Usage:

1. Mix oils together and use to massage the affected area. Use upward motions.

2. Repeat 2 to 3 times every day.

ESSENTIAL OILS FOR PAINS IN THE BODY

Essential Oil Liniment For Joint Pain

Several factors cause joint pain. They include: injury, overuse and damage from previous injury or disease. The condition may be mild, lasting for a few hours or it may be chronic, lasting for several years. Essential oil helps to limit the inflammation that often comes with it.

Eucalyptus essential oil - 8 drops

Peppermint essential oil - 8 drops

Rosemary essential oil -   8 drops

Cinnamon leaf oil - 4 drops

Juniper berry oil - 4 drops

Marjoram essential oil - 4 drops

Vegetable oil or Alcohol (either rubbing or vodka) - 2 ounces

Usage:

1. Mix ingredients. Stir a few times every day for three days to disperse the oils in the alcohol.

2. This formula must be used only on the painful joints because it is stronger than the typical massage oil so it mustn't be used over a large area of the body. Use several times daily as needed.

Cramp Relief EO For Muscle Pain

Muscles may hurt after a long day of work or vigorous exercise. Repeated daily activities may also tighten muscles, causing them to cramp.

Lavender essential oil - 12 drops

Marjoram essential Oil - 6 drops

Chamomile essential Oil - 4 drops

Ginger essential oil - 4 drops

Vegetable oil - 2 ounces

Usage:

1. Combine all ingredients. Apply daily over the cramping area as often as needed

Nerve Pain Essential Oil Treatment

Damaged nerves can be quite painful because the nerves register pain. Injured nerves also take a long time to regenerate. However, essential oil helps with the treatment process. They relieve pain and speed up healing.

Chamomile essential oil - 4 drops

Marjoram essential oil - 3 drops

Helichrysum oil (optional) - 3 drops

Lavender oil - 2 drops

Vegetable oil - 1 ounce

Usage:

Combine all the ingredients. For pain relief, apply as needed all through the day.

Arthritic Soaking Bath Blend

Bath Salt Blend 1-2 cups

Lavender essential oil - 2 drops

Rosemary essential oil - 2 drops

Juniper berry essential oil - 4 drops

Cypress essential oil - 2 drops

Usage:

Add this blend to bath and soak for 20 to 30 minutes.

Rheumatic Pain Essential Oil Blend

Lavender Essential Oil - 2 drops

Ginger Essential Oil- 4 drops

Silver Fir Essential Oil- 4 drops

Carrier oil of choice- 4 teaspoons

Usage:

Combine and apply on affected areas.

Massage Blend For Sore Joints/ Arthritis

Coriander essential oil - 3 drops

Roman Chamomile essential oil - 6 drops

Black Pepper essential oil - 1 drop

Marjoram essential oil - 4 drops

Rosemary essential oil - 3 drops

Ginger essential oil - 1 drop

Carrier Oil of choice - 2 ounces

Usage:

1. Blend well and store in a plastic bottle.

2. Massage daily into sore joints.

Achy Muscle Soother
Lemongrass essential oil – 2 drops

Ginger essential oil - 4 drops

Lavender essential oil - 4 drops

Almond oil - 4 teaspoons

Usage:

Combine and apply on affected areas.

Tendonitis Relief With Essential Oil
Tendonitis is simply the inflammation of a tendon. While overuse is the main cause of this often painful and debilitating condition, it can also be brought about by infection or rheumatic disease.

Knee, ankle, wrist or Achilles tendonitis along with the elbow, foot and wrist pain that comes with them are difficult to treat. However, natural essentials oils can offer a measure of relief and quicken the healing process.

Basil essential oil -10 drops

Wintergreen essential oil - 8 drops

Cypress essential oil - 6 drops

Peppermint essential oil - 3 drops

Usage:

1. Mix oils together, rub on location. Can also be mixed with 2 tbsp of jojoba oil and massage larger areas of the body.

ESSENTIAL OIL RECIPES FOR SKIN BLEMISHES/COSMETIC PROBLEMS

Aromatherapy Treatment For Acne
It's ok to have one or two pimples now and then but when breakouts are frequent; this blend can be very helpful.

Geranium essential oil - 3 drops

Tea Tree or Lemongrass essential oil - 7 drops

Lavender essential oil - 10 drops

Jojoba oil or Aloe Vera gel - 30ml

Usage:

1. Mix jojoba oil with essential oils in a dark glass bottle.

2. Apply a little quantity to affected areas of the skin twice a day. Avoid eyes, lips and nose.

3. Results will appear if used consistently for a few weeks.

Relief For Prickly Heat Rash In Children

Use this combination for babies two years and under. Older children will require double the measurement.

Lavender essential oil - 2 drops

Baking Soda - 1/4 cup

Usage:

1. Mix the two ingredients together then add to bath water.

Itchy Skin Recipe

Lavender essential oil - 5 drops

Tea Tree essential oil - 3 drops

Frankincense essential oil - 2 drops

Witch hazel - 2 ounces

Usage:

1. Fill a 2 ounce spray bottle halfway with witch hazel, add the essential oils, shake together then fill remaining space with witch hazel.

2. Apply this mixture on itchy skin.

Remedy For Liver Spots (Age Spots)
Frankincense essential oil - 2 drops

Lavender essential oil - 2 drops

Myrrh essential oil - 2 drops

Extra virgin coconut oil - 10ml

Usage:

1. Mix the ingredients together and apply topical at least once a day.

Dark circles Or Bags Under Eyes
Roman Chamomile essential oil - 1 drop

Lavender essential oil - 1 drop

Aloe Vera gel or other lotion/cream - 30mls

Usage:

1. Mix the essential oils properly with aloe vera gel.

2. Once a day, cleanse and dry the face then rub the blend very gently below and above the eye socket.

3. Avoid contact with eyelids or eyelashes so you will not get some in your eyes.

Healing Blend For Chapped Lips

Geranium essential oil - 2 drops

Chamomile essential oil - 1 drop

Rose essential oil - 2 drops

Neroli essential oil - 1 drop

Aloe Vera oil - 20 ml

Usage:

1. Mix and apply this blend to chapped lips for healing and pain relief.

Treatment For Cracked Skin

The Lavender oil in this blend will help to fight infected cracks in the skin. You should also endeavor to drink adequate water daily to keep your body hydrated.

Lavender essential oil - 10 drops

Helichrysum essential oil - 5 drops

Neroli essential oil - 5 drops

Lotion - 1 ounce

Usage:

1. Mix the essential oils with 1 ounce of your body lotion and apply as many times as necessary daily. It will stimulate healing of cracks and the regeneration of new cells.

Dry Skin Moisturizer

Geranium essential oil - 7 drops

Sandalwood essential oil - 10 drops

Rosewood essential oil - 3 drops

Ylang Ylang essential oil - 5 drops

Carrier oil - 2 ounces

Usage:

1. Mix all ingredients together in a bottle.

2. Apply 4 - 6 drops of this blend to dry area twice a day.

Oily Skin Remedy

Geranium essential oil - 3 drops

Grapefruit essential oil - 3 drops

Lavender essential oil - 3 drops

Evening primrose carrier oil - 30ml

Usage:

1. Mix the ingredients in a glass bottle and apply a little quantity to your face every day.

Oily Skin And Acne Steam Bath

This recipe is good for stimulating facial skin.

Lemon essential oil - 4 drops

Juniper Berry essential oil - 6 drops

Cypress essential oil - 4 drops

Usage:

1. Add the oils above to a bowl of hot water.

2. Bend over the bowl; drape a towel over your head and the bowl to prevent the escape of steam.

3. Hold this position for 5-10 minutes then use tepid water to rinse your face and pat dry.

Skin Firming Remedy For Flabby Skin

If your skin is sagging after weight loss, the usage of aromatherapy oils can restore elasticity and improve blood flow.

Patchouli essential oil - 8 drops

Cypress essential oil - 5 drops

Geranium essential oil - 5 drops

Sandalwood essential oil - 1 drop

Jojoba oil - 1/2 teaspoon

Usage:

1. Mix these ingredients together to make a soothing skin serum.

2. Massage affected areas before bed at night and sometimes in the morning.

Stretch Marks Treatment Lotion

Lavender essential oil - 3 drops

Frankincense essential oil - 3 drops

Geranium essential oil - 3 drops

Helichrysum essential oil - 3 drops

Virgin coconut oil - 1 ounce

Usage:

1. Use this blend as body lotion on affected areas.

Stretch Marks Cocoa Butter Cream
Neroli essential oil - 4 drops

Cocoa butter (deodorized) - 3 ounces

Avocado oil - 1 ounce

Usage:

1. Melt cocoa butter in a double boiler then stir in avocado oil.

2. Pour the mixture in a bowl to cool then add the essential oil.

3. Transfer to a 4 ounce jar with a lid and use as body cream.

4. Store in the refrigerator to avoid the growth of mold.

Wrinkles And Mature Skin Blend
Frankincense - 5 drops

Lavender - 15 drops

Carrot seed - 5 drops

Neroli - 5 drops

Jojoba oil - 2 ounces

Usage:

1. Mix ingredients together in a dark bottle.

2. Massage the affected areas as needed.

Sun Spots Aromatherapy Remedy

Frankincense essential oil - 5 drops

Lavender essential oil - 5 drops

Distilled water

Usage:

1. Mix these essential oils with water in a 2 ounce spray bottle.

2. Spray this mixture on your skin before rubbing on your sunscreen or moisturizer every other day.

Sunburn Spray Soother

Lavender oil - 20 drops

Aloe Vera juice - 4 ounces

200 IU vitamin E oil

Vinegar - 1 tablespoon

Usage:

1. Combine all the ingredients. Place in a spritzer bottle. Shake well before using as often as needed.

2. Keeping the spray refrigerated provides extra relief due to the coolness.

Sunscreen Recipe

Helichrysum essential oil - 30 drops

Lavender essential oil - 30 drops

Fractionated Coconut oil

Usage

1. Add the essential oils to 2 ounce spray bottle then fill up the bottle with fractionated coconut oil.

2. Shake and spray on your body as sunscreen.

Aromatherapy For Scars
Scars can develop from scrapes, cuts or surgery. You can reduce the visibility of these blemishes with the use of essential oils.

Helichrysum essential oil - 6 drops

Lavender essential oil - 4 drops

Rosehip seed oil - 1 ounce

Usage:

1. Mix this combination in a bottle.

2. Start using daily on the cut once it is sealed shut (this could be after a few days). Apply the blend over the scab and the immediate area. Do not remove the scabs on the surface. Picking or removing scabs will lead to scarring.

3. If you had a surgery, start applying the blend once the staples and sutures are removed.

4. This blend can also be used on old scars but it takes 3-6 months to get results.

ESSENTIAL OIL HAIR CARE

Remedy For Light Dandruff
Dandruff occurs when excessive skin oils and cells die and flake off in unusually large quantities. Although not a serious condition, it is often embarrassing.

Melaleuca -2 to 3 drops

Any high quality shampoo

Usage

Add oil to shampoo and use.

Essential Oil Blend For Heavy Dandruff
Any carrier oil - 1 teaspoon

Lemon essential oil - 4 drops

Lavender essential oil - 4 drops

Melaleuca essential oil- 4 drops

Rosemary essential oil- 4 drops

Usage

Massage blend into the scalp every night. Cover with shower cap. Shampoo it out the following morning.

Essential Oil To Prevent Flaking From Harsh Hair Products

Break the cycle of damaged scalp and flaking caused by substandard dandruff shampoos by using the following:

Birch, Wintergreen or Rosemary - 4 -6 drops

Shampoo - 1/2 ounce

Usage

1. Mix oil into shampoo. Apply1 inch partings in the hair and then rub mixture into scalp.

2. Leave on for 5-7 minutes and then apply regular shampoo and conditioning.

Mild Hair Loss Remedy

Mix together 1 - 2 drops of Rosemary essential oil to shampoo

Use it every day to stimulate follicle

Serious Hair Loss Remedy

Rosemary essential oil - 3 drops

Lavender essential oil - 5 drops

Cypress essential oil - 4 drops

Clary Sage essential oil - 4 drops

Sandalwood - 10 drops

Usage:

Combine all ingredients and pour in your hair shampoo.

ESSENTIAL OIL RECIPES FOR SKIN PROBLEMS

Aromatherapy Treatment Of Boils
Boils can appear on different parts of the body and can sometimes be associated with fever and fatigue.

Tea tree essential oil - 2 drops

Lavender essential oil - 2 drops

Juniper essential oil - 1 drop

Usage:

1. Dilute the essential oils in 200 ml of hot water.

2. Bathe the infected area twice daily with this mixture.

3. 1drop of Chamomile essential oil should be added if there is severe inflammation.

Ringworm Treatment
The Melaleuca and Thyme in this blend are effective against fungal infections while the Lavender will aid healing of the skin.

Melaleuca essential oil - 30 drops

Thyme essential oil - 30 drops

Lavender essential oil - 30 drops

Usage:

1. Apply 2-3 drops of this combination topically on infected area 3 times daily for 10 to 12 days

Eczema And Dermatitis Treatment
This blend will relieve itching, sooth the skin and also stimulate healing.

Helichrysum essential oil - 5 drops

Melaleuca essential oil- 3 drops

Lavender essential oil - 10 drops

Myrrh essential oil - 5 drops

Extra virgin coconut oil - 1 teaspoon

Usage:

1. Mix together and apply topically on affected area daily.

Scabies Aromatherapy Treatment
Peppermint essential oil - 4 drops

Lavender essential oil - 4 drops

Sweet Almond oil - 1 teaspoon

Usage:

1. Apply this blend to itching areas 2-3 times a day, after a bath.

2. Wash clothing of affected person at high temperature. Spray pillows, mattresses, couches with a mixture of 5% lavender, 5% white camphor and 90% alcohol. Wear a mask while spraying to avoid inhaling.

Remedy For Warts

Lemon essential oil - 12 drops

Bergamot FCF essential oil - 4 drops

Tea Tree essential oil - 4 drops

Cypress essential oil - 3 drops

Thyme essential oil - 4 drops

Jojoba oil - 1 tablespoon

Usage:

1. Blend together in a dark glass bottle.

2. Apply 2 drops of this blend to the wart then cover with a Band-Aid.

3. Do this once a day for 2 weeks.

Note: Use 2 teaspoons of jojoba oil if using on the elderly or children.

Shingles Relief With Essential Oil

Shingles is a skin rash caused by an inflammation of the nerve and skin. It is caused by the same virus that causes chicken-pot.

Melaleuca essential oil - 30 drops

Eucalyptus essential oil - 30 drops

Lavender essential oil - 30 drops

Usage:

1. Mix and add to a 4-ounce spray bottle. Fill it with fractionated coconut oil. Shake thoroughly before spraying.

2. Spray directly to affected area as often as needed to deal with the pain.

Bed Sores (Pressure Ulcers)

Bedsores or pressure ulcers are injuries that often develop from continuous pressure applied to the skin when in a limited area. People who are confined to a chair or bed for an extended period usually experience this problem.

Lavender essential oil- 10 drops

Helichrysum essential oil -6 drops

Myrrh essential oil -6 drops

Geranium essential oil -4 drops

Melaleuca essential oil -4 drops

2 tbs. FCO or EVCO carrier oil

Usage:

Apply topically thrice a day

Emergency Burn Wash/Compress

While Second and third degree burns call for immediate medical attention, first degree burns as well as sunburns can be subdued by essential oils. Essential oils also provide protection from bacterial infection that usually occurs with burns.

Lavender oil- 5 drops

Water - 1 pint, about 50°F

Usage:

1. Add essential oil to water, stirring thoroughly to disperse the oil.

2. Dip the burned area in the water for a few minutes. Alternatively, soak a soft cloth in the water and apply to burned area. Leave the compress on for 15-20 minutes then soak again and reapply 2-3 times more.

ESSENTIAL OILS FOR INSECT AND ANIMAL BITES

Essential Oil For Gnat And Chigger Bites

Although bites and stings from insects such as mosquitoes and ants produce a lot of discomfort, including redness and swelling, they can easily be dealt with.

However, bites from insects like scorpions and black widow are usually very harmful and must seriously be attended to. In both cases, essential oil can provide a measure of relief.

Cider vinegar - 1 teaspoon

Thyme essential oil - 3 drops

Usage:

1. Clean bitten area with warm soapy water, rinse and dry.

2. Combine the oil and vinegar and dab on affected area for relief.

Mosquito &Other Minor Insect Bites

Lavender, peppermint or tea tree essential oil - 1-3 drops

Usage:

1. For relief from itching, dab oil topically on affected area.

2. Repeat every 1-2 hours if necessary.

3. For very sensitive skin and for young children, dilute essential oil with a carrier oil

4. Note: Chamomile essential oils can reduce swelling and inflammation

Dog Bite Relief Blend

If there is no broken skin, clean the area and apply 1-2 drops of Melaleuca topically.

1. for puncture wound:

- Clean the area and apply 1 to 2 drops of Frankincense topically.

-Dilute with carrier oil so the oils can penetrate easily into the puncture.

- Bandage and treat twice per day for 2 to 3 days.

2. for open wounds with torn flesh:

-Stop the bleeding using Helichrysum and pressure.

-Clean the area and then topically apply Melaleuca and frankincense.

3. Note:

-If skin is damaged to the point where stitches are required or there is danger of damaged bones, tendons, ligaments or nerves, seek immediate professional medical assistance.

-Additionally, if there is risk of rabies, the animal should be captured if possible.

Essential Oil To Repel Bugs

Lemon essential oil - 19 drops

Cajeput essential oil - 25 drops

Cedarwood essential oil - 13 drops

Geranium essential oil - 19 drops

Sweet almond oil - 2 oz

Usage:

1. Mix all the essential oils in a recyclable Plastic bottle.

2. Add the almond oil and Shake until thoroughly blended.

3. Apply thinly to exposed skin as needed.

Remedy For Bee Stings &Serious Insect Bites

1. Remove the stinger first.

2. Then apply lavender or roman chamomile as above.

3. Apply a cold compress over bitten area, changing regularly.

4. Do NOT use ice as it could cause damage to the skin if it becomes accidentally frozen.

5. Seek immediate medical assistance if allergic to bee stings or others.

ESSENTIAL OIL FOR ORAL HEALTH

EO Simple Mouth Wash

Peppermint essential oil - 2 drops

Lemon essential oil - 4 drops

Distilled water- 2 cups

Usage:

1. Add oils to water. Shake thoroughly before each use.

2. Swish a mouthful for 1 to 2 minutes and spit out.

Gum Essential Oil Blend

Tea Tree essential oil - 10 drops

Peppermint essential oil - 1 drop

Lemon essential oil - 3 drops

Myrrh essential oil - 6 drops

Almond oil - 1 teaspoon

Usage:

1. After brushing the teeth and rinsing the mouth with mouthwash, combine the above oils and apply a small quantity on your gums daily.

2. Consult your dentist if the gums or the source of irritation do not heal.

Therapeutic Fresh Breath Mouthwash
Tea Tree essential oil - 2 drops

Myrrh essential oil - 2 drops

Peppermint essential oil - 1 drop

Distilled water - 4 to 8 Ounces

Usage:

1. Mix together in a glass or plastic PET bottle. Shake well before use.

2. Swish about 1/2 ounce in your mouth after eating as required or after brushing your teeth.

Throat Gargle/Spray For Sore Throat
Marjoram essential oil - 4 drops

Warm water - 1/2 cup

Salt - 1/2 teaspoon

Usage:

1. Combine the ingredients.

2. Shake thoroughly to disperse the oils and dissolve the salt before spraying or gargling.

3. Gargle every 30 minutes initially and then several times daily.

Neck Wrap Remedy For Sore Throat
Sore throat may be caused by bacterial infection, yelling, lots of talking or singing. Sometimes, the throat may be so inflamed that swallowing will be difficult.

Lavender essential oil - 2 drops

51

Bergamot essential oil - 2 drops

Tea tree essential oil - 1 drop

Hot water - 2 cups

Usage:

1. Mix essential oils with water. Soak a flannel in the still warm water, wring it out.

2. Wrap around neck and then cover with a thin towel to retain the heat. Take it off before it becomes cold. Use all through the day as frequently as you desire.

Toothache Oil Blend
Clove bud essential oil - 4 drops

Orange essential oil (for flavor) - 1 drop

Vegetable oil - 1 teaspoon

Usage:

1. Combine ingredients and then rub a few drops onto the painful gums. Repeat frequently.

2. Put clove bud in the most painful area of the mouth during an emergency. Gently mash the clove with the teeth as it softens. This way, the oil is released and you can then suck on it.

3. Some young children may find clove oil too hot for them. You can replace it with chamomile oil. Since chamomile is less effective as a pain killer, apply treatment as frequently as possible.

Tonsillitis Essential Oil Relief

Tonsillitis simply means inflammation of the tonsils. It is generally caused by viral or bacterial infection. It may be treated via different medical procedures but essential oil basically helps to lessen the swelling and discomfort.

Water - 1 qt

Lemon, lavender or eucalyptus essential oil - 3 drops

Usage:

1. Boil water and add the essential oils. Place toweled head over hot pot of water. Breathe the aroma.

2. May also be drank as tea to relieve sore throat or used in a warm bath.

Bad Breath Due To Digestive Issues

Peppermint essential oil - 2 drops

Lemon essential oil - 2 drops

Brandy - a teaspoon

Bad Breath Due To Gum Disease

Tea tree essential oil - 2 drops

Thyme essential oil - 2 drops

Usage For Both Recipes

1. Dilute the essential oil in brandy. Add mixture to a glass of warm water.

2. Sip, swirl around then mouth and spit out. Do not swallow.

Remedy For Mouth Ulcers (Stomatitis)

Mouth ulcers also called Stomatitis or canker sores mostly occur on the tongue, inner lip, inner cheek, floor of the mouth and soft palate.

The condition is usually painful, making it difficult to eat and chew. It is caused by a variety of factors including dietary deficiencies, Candida and friction from a denture.

Myrrh essential oil - 3 drops

Alcohol - 1 teaspoon

Usage:

1. Using a cotton-bud, dab directly onto the ulcer. (May sting for a while but is often very effective).

2. Alternatively, dilute with half a glass of water and make into a mouthwash.

Mouth Alcer Treatment For Children

Myrrh essential oil is extremely bitter especially for children so it is best to add Peppermint, mandarin or Fennel oil to this mixture.

Myrrh essential oil - 2 drops

Peppermint essential oil - 1 drop

Alcohol - 1 teaspoon

Usage:

1. Using a cotton-bud, dab directly onto the ulcer.

2. Alternatively, dilute with half a glass of water and make into a mouthwash.

ESSENTIAL OIL FOR FOOT AND LEG CARE

Simple Foot Powder Blend
Thyme essential oil - 2 drops

Tea Tree essential oil - 2 drops

Rosemary essential oil - 5 drops

Talc Powder - 5 oz

Usage:

1. Place oils in powder. Shake thoroughly and let it sit for 24 hours. Before using on your feet, shake again. Use daily.

2. Dust on your feet after showering. Be sure to spread your toes.

Essential Oil Preparation For Dry Cracked Heels
Geranium essential oil - 10 drops

Melaleuca essential oil- 10 drops

Peppermint essential oil -10 drops

Virgin Coconut Oils - 1 tablespoon

Usage:

1. Blend together. Apply topically on area every morning and evening.

2. Cover with socks

Food Bath Blend (for tired feet)

Grapefruit essential oil - 4 drops

Myrtle essential oil - 4 drops

Cajeput essential oil - 3 drops

Spearmint essential oil - 4 drops

Sesame, Almond or Hazelnut carrier oil -1 teaspoon

Usage:

1. Blend all ingredients and add to a basin of warm water. Swirl around and then soak in your feet.

2. Relax for about 15 minutes.

Remedy For Foot Odor

Lavender- 2-3 drops

Basin of lukewarm water

Usage:

1. Add oil to bath and then place feet (safe for blistered and cracked feet as well) in it for 10- 15 minutes.

Essential Oil Blend For Calluses And Corns

Although calluses are generally painless, they tend to be painful on the bottom of feet where they occur due to poorly fitting shoes. Corns occur above the toe joints and they can cause a lot of discomfort as well.

Myrrh essential oil - 6 drops

Vanilla essential oil - 4 drops

Lavender essential oil - 12 drops

Sweet almond - 2 ounces

Usage:

1. Mix together in a bottle, shaking well to mix.

2. Massage into the affected area to soften calluses and corns. Apply daily.

Anti-Fungus Blend For Athletic Foot

Sweaty feet that are cloistered in socks and shoes are the leading cause of Athlete's foot. Such moist environments attract fungus.

Tea tree essential oil - 12 drops

Geranium essential oil   8 drops

Thyme essential oil - 3 drops

Tincture of benzoin - 1 tablespoon

Apple cider vinegar - 2 ounces

Myrrh essential oil - 2 drops (optional)

Usage:

1. Combine all ingredients. Shake well before use.

2. Use as wash daily or as often as needed or dab on afflicted area.

Athletic Foot Fungal Powder

Lemon eucalyptus or tea tree essential oil - 14 drops

Geranium essential oil - 8 drops

Sage essential oil - 5 drops

Peppermint essential oil - 1 drop

Cornstarch - 1/4 cup

Usage:

1. Place the cornstarch in a plastic bag. Gently sprinkle in the essential oils, evenly distributing them through the powder.

2. Next, close the bag and then toss the powder. This will break up any formed clumps. Store the powder in a glass or ceramic container or a sealed plastic bag. A perforated lidded shake bottle will even make dispensing easier to achieve. Use powder once daily or as often as needed

Gout Relief Blend

This blend is effective for the common gout that comes with intense pain and redness of the big toe.

Frankincense essential oil 10 drops

Basil essential oil - 10 drops

Usage:

1. Mix the oils together in a dark bottle.

2. Apply 2-3 drops of the blend to the painful area then cover with hot compress.

3. Repeat 2 or 3 times per day.

ESSENTIAL OIL FOR CUTS, BRUISES & BONES

Balm Relief For Minor Cuts& Scrapes

Minor cuts are scrapes are inevitable. This balm recipe prepares you for immediate aromatherapy treatment when one is needed.

Lavender essential oil - 40 drops

Tea Tree essential oil - 40 drops

Grated Beeswax - 1 ounce

Vegetable carrier oil (Jojoba, Sweet Almond Oil) - 3 ounces

Wide-mouth jar - 4 ounce

Usage:

1. In a double boiler, heat the beeswax at low setting. In a separate pan, slowly heat your carrier oil. Next, pour the heated carrier into a medium bowl. Add the melted beeswax, stirring thoroughly.

2. Add lavender and tea tree essential oils, stirring well again. Pour this mixture into a wide-mouth jar. Leave to cool for about 5-10 minutes before tightening with the lid. Wait until cooled before using.

3. To use: clean the minor cuts and scrapes and then apply a thin amount of the balm. Bandage if necessary.

Germ Fighter Spray *(to prevent infection and foster healing)*

Tea tree essential oil -12 drops

Eucalyptus essential oil - 6 drops

Lemon essential oil - 6 drops

Distilled water - 2 ounces

Usage:

Combine ingredients. Dispense formula from a spray bottle. Before each use, shake well to disperse the oils.

Essential Oil Blend For Bruises
As anti-inflammatory oil, Helichrysum essential oil is remarkable and helps to ease the discomfort and unsightliness of bruising.

Helichrysum essential oil - 8 drops

Jojoba or sweet almond oil- 1 ounce

Usage:

1. Combine both oils, mixing well.

2. Store in a dark colored glass bottle.

Pain Relief Blend *(To calm the wounded)*

Lavender essential –2 or 3 drops

Usage:

Apply directly to wound. Put also on the palms, rub together and inhale the oil's calming fragrance.

Essential Oil Blend For Bone Spurs

Bone spurs (osteophytes) is simply an added bone growth to a normal bone area. This condition usually occurs after an injury as the body attempts to repair itself. Common activities like running, dancing and even wearing tight shoes can cause bone spurs.

Wintergreen essential oil - 4 drops

Eucalyptus essential oil - 4 drops

Marjoram essential oil - 4 drops

Cypress essential oil - 4 drops

Helichrysum essential oil - 4 drops

Peppermint essential oil - 4 drops

Frankincense essential oil - 4 drops

Coconut oil carrier - 10 drops

Usage:

1. Mix ingredients and apply to affected area twice daily until the bone spur gone.

2. Continue for more 2 weeks. Wrap with a warm cloth to speed up results and then wrap with plastic bag and extra towel to keep heat in.

Alternative Bone Spur Solution

Eucalyptus essential oil - 5 drops

Marjoram essential oil - 5 drops

Cypress essential oil -   5 drops

Lavender essential oil - 5 drops

Thyme essential oil -   5 drops

Basil essential oil -   5 drops

Coconut carrier oil - 30 drops

<u>Usage:</u>

1. Mix ingredients and apply to affected area twice daily until the bone spur gone.

2. Continue for more 2 weeks. Wrap with a warm cloth to speed up results and then wrap with plastic bag and extra towel to keep heat in. Reported results took between 2 weeks to 3 months.

Remedy For Broken Bones

Broken or fractured bones can happen anywhere in the body. Here are the essential oils that will help:

- For pain relief: Wintergreen essential oil

- For stress relief: Lavender essential oil

- For healing: Birch essential oil (bone repair), Helichrysum (nerve damage, overall tissue regeneration and repair), Cypress (circulation), Lemongrass essential oil (ligaments), White Fir (anti-inflammatory) and Marjoram (tissue rebuilding).

<u>Usage:</u>

1. Apply 1-2 drops topically to injured area 2- 3 times daily.

ESSENTIAL OIL RECIPES FOR EMOTIONAL HEALTH

Alertness And Energizing Blend
Use this blend when you have demanding tasks ahead of you and you want to be mentally alert and aware.

Juniper essential oil - 14 drops

Rosemary essential oil - 8 drops

Pine needle essential oil - 8 drops

Usage:

1. Blend all the ingredients in a dark bottle.

2. Place several drops in your home, office or car diffuser (for long distance driving).

3. When diffusing in the car, use only for 20 minutes at a time.

Anxiety Relief Recipe
It is not always possible to avoid things that make you anxious. You can however handle uncertainties better when you use nerve-calming essential oils.

Geranium essential oil - 2 drops

Vanilla essential oil - 2 drops

Neroli essential oil - 3 drops

Rosewood essential oil - 2 drops

Frankincense essential oil - 1 drop

Ylang ylang essential oil - 2 drops

Rose essential oil - 1 drop

Usage:

1. Mix properly in dark glass bottle.

2. Use in a nasal inhaler or just place 1-2 drops on tissue or cotton ball and inhale.

Romantic Massage Blend

Several essential oils can enhance the feeling of excitement and stimulate sensations for romantic encounters.

Orange essential oil - 2 drops

Jasmine essential oil - 2 drops

Ylang ylang essential oil - 1 drop

Sandalwood essential oil - 2 drops

Almond oil - 1 ounce

Usage:

1. Mix the ingredients properly.

2. Use for a slow and loving, romantic massage.

Aphrodisiac For Love And Romance

Sandalwood essential oil - 3 drops

Rose essential oil - 2 drops

Lotion - 1 or 2 tablespoons

Usage:

1. Mix the essential oils into 1 or 2 tablespoons of your body lotion.

2. Apply on your arms, face and body.

Aromatherapy For Burnout, Exhaustion & Fatigue
These oils can rejuvenate and lift you up when you have been through a physically and mentally exhaustive circumstance.

Lime essential oil - 15 drops

Grapefruit essential oil - 8 drops

Cardamom essential oil - 8 drop

Usage:

1. Add a few drops into a diffuser in the room where you are resting.

2. Mix with 2 ounces of almond oil and treat yourself to a relaxing massage to release tense muscles.

Note: Exhaustion and burnout will require several days of adequate rest and sleep.

Seasonal Affective Disorder (SAD)& Cabin Fever
It is natural for some people to have the blues for one or two days when the seasons are changing.

Geranium essential oil - 15 drops

Bergamot essential oil - 10 drops

Lavender essential oil - 5 drops

Usage:

1. Blend the oils together and use in a diffuser.

2. Add 6-8 drops of this blend to the bath tub and soak in the water.

Note: Endeavor to go outside within the daylight hours to make you feel better during this time.

Concentration Enhancing Blend
Lemon essential oil - 20 drops

Basil essential oil - 6 drops

Rosemary essential oil - 2 drops

Usage:

1. Mix these essential oils together then diffuse into the air.

2. If you are at work, you can place a personal diffuser on your desk or just put a few drops of the blend on tissue for inhaling.

Confidence Booster
When you feel confident, it is easier to tackle tasks and challenges more effectively. This blend will give you the needed emotional support to strengthen your confidence.

Orange essential oil - 10 drops

Grapefruit essential oil - 10 drops

Bergamot essential oil - 5 drops

Usage:

1. Mix the oils together and use several drops in an inhaler.

Confidence Boosting Rub
Rosemary essential oil - 20 drops

Fennel essential oil - 10 drops

Carrier oil or lotion - 2 ounces

Usage:

1. Mix together the ingredients and apply to your skin when needed.

Happiness Enhancing Blend

Although essential oils cannot create happiness, they can help to clear your mind so you can focus on things that make you happy. Use the following blend to bring up your spirits.

Rose geranium essential oil - 5 drops

Orange essential oil - 19 drops

Cinnamon essential oil - 1 drop

Clove essential oil - 1 drop

Usage:

1. Blend these oils and use in a diffuser.

2. Use 5 drops in your bath.

Comfort For Grief& Loss

It is natural to go through a period of grief when you lose a loved one, a job or a pet. Essential oils can help with the sorrow and sadness being experienced at this time.

Vanilla essential oil - 5 drops

Mandarin essential oil - 3 drops

Rose Otto essential oil - 3 drops

Roman Chamomile essential oil - 3 drops

Usage:

1. Blend the oils in a dark glass bottle and use in your diffuser.

2. Blend oils with 1 ounce of Almond or Jojoba oil and use for massage.

Insomnia Sleep Time Blend

In addition to using this blend, you should also avoid stimulating foods like coffee, colas and some teas in the evening and also avoid stimulating entertainment (movies or talk shows) close to bedtime.

Sandalwood essential oil - 6 drops

Ylang Ylang essential oil - 2 drops

Neroli essential oil - 2 drops

Vetiver essential oil - 1 drop

Coriander essential oil - 1 drop

Jojoba oil - 1 tablespoon

Usage:

1. Blend essential oils with Jojoba.

2. Take a warm bath before bedtime then apply this blend to pulse points such as inside of the wrists, behind the ears and behind the knees.

Insomnia Massage Blend

Marjoram essential oil - 1 drop

Ylang Ylang essential oil - 1 drop

Roman Chamomile essential oil - 1 drop

Sweet Orange essential oil - 1 drop

Tangerine essential oil - 1 drop

Lavender essential oil - 1 drop

Carrier oil - 1 ounce

Usage:

1. Mix the oils together and massage your body at bedtime.

Memory Loss Recovery Blend

Memory loss is predominant in the elderly but it can also be experienced occasionally by younger people. Essential oils like Rosemary and Basil are used for dementia and Alzheimer's patients in many nursing facilities.

Basil essential oil - 6 drops

Lemon essential oil - 20 drops

Rosemary essential oil - 2 drops

Usage:

1. Mix the oils together and use in a diffuser.

Nervousness And Anxiety

Here is a useful anti-anxiety blend.

Lavender essential oil - 10 drops

Orange essential oil -10 drops

Marjoram essential oil - 2 drops

Cedarwood essential oil - 2 drops

Sweet Almond oil - 4 ounces

Usage:

1. Combine ingredients in a small glass bottle.

2. Open and inhale whenever you feel nervous.

Stress Eliminating Recipe

Lavender essential oil - 15 drops

Lemon essential oil - 10 drops

Clary Sage essential oil - 5 drops

Usage:

1. Mix together in an amber bottle.

2. Use in a diffuser or personal nasal inhaler.

3. Add 5-6 drops of this blend to warm bath water and soak in it for 20-30 minutes.

Positive Energy Recipe

Orange essential oil - 4 drops

Lavender essential oil - 3 drops

Rose essential oil - 1or 2 drops

Usage:

1. Add these essential oils to 2 ounces of distilled water in a spray bottle.

2. Spray often in your work area.

Overcoming Insecurity

Essential oils can help to enhance self confidence and strengthen your emotions when you are feeling insecure.

Bergamot essential oil - 2 drops

Cedarwood essential oil - 2 drops

Frankincense essential oil - 1 drop

Usage:

1. Multiply this recipe by 4 to make 20 drops. Keep in a dark glass bottle then use the necessary number of drops in a diffuser.

2. For bath oil, multiply this recipe by 3 to make 15 drops then mix with 2 ounces of Jojoba oil in a dark glass bottle. Use 1-2 teaspoonfuls per bath.

Loneliness Diffuser Blend

This blend is helpful when you feel lonely.

Bergamot essential oil - 8 drops

Frankincense essential oil - 8 drops

Rose essential oil - 4 drops

Usage:

1. Mix together properly in a dark bottle.

2. Use appropriate drops in a diffuser.

Loneliness Bath Oil

Bergamot essential oil - 6 drops

Frankincense essential oil - 6 drops

Rose essential oil - 3 drop

Jojoba oil - 2 ounces

Usage:

1. Blend oils together in a dark glass bottle.

2. Use 1-2 teaspoonfuls in your bath water.

Panic& Panic Attacks Diffuser Blend
Use this blend in times of panic.

Lavender essential oil - 16 drops

Rose essential oil - 4 drops

Usage:

1. Add oils to a dark glass bottle and shake together.

2. Use this blend in your diffuser.

Panic &Panic Attacks Bath Oil
Lavender essential oil - 12 drops

Rose essential oil - 3 drops

Jojoba oil - 2 ounces

Usage:

1. Mix essential oils with Jojoba in a dark glass bottle.

2. Add 1-2 teaspoons to your bath water.

Emotional Shock Relief

Emotional shock can occur when you hear bad news or experience a negative occurrence.

The following essential oils can help you to calm down until normalcy returns.

Lavender

Neroli

Tea Tree

Rose

Roman Chamomile

Usage:

1. Keep a vial of any of these oils in a purse or pocket.

2. Place a few drops on tissue or cotton ball and inhale. You could also use a nasal inhaler.

3. Mix any of the oils with a little carrier oil for a back rub or foot rub.

ESSENTIAL OILS FOR WOMEN ISSUES

Vaginitis (Virginal Inflammation)

This condition is mostly caused by a bacteria and very rarely fungal infection. 75% of women will experience this condition in their lifetime.

Lavender and Melaleuca- 2 - 5 drops each

Extra Virgin Coconut Oil- 1 tablespoon (1/2 ounce)

Usage:

Add essential oils to coconut oil. Soak into a tampon. Use nightly for a week

Mood Soother For PMS

PMS is the acronym for premenstrual syndrome. It comprises various symptoms that generally begin several days before menstruation.

These symptoms include breast swelling and tenderness, water retention, depression, irritability, headaches and mood swings.

Geranium essential oil - 9 drops

Chamomile essential oil - 6 drops

Clary sage essential oil - 3 drops

Angelica essential oil (if available) - 3 drops

Marjoram essential oil - 2 drops

Vegetable essential oil - 2 ounces

Usage:

1. Combine all ingredients. The angelica oil works real well but it is optional because it may be hard to find.

2. Add 1- 2 teaspoons to bath or use as massage oil. For more effectiveness, add 1- 2 drops of neroli, jasmine or rose. Without the vegetable oil, it can be used in a diffuser or place in a vial to smell as needed.

Bloating & Headache Relief Blend

Lavender essential oil - 6 drops

Juniper berry essential oil - 3 drops

Birch essential oil - 2 drops

Patchouli essential oil (optional) - 1 drop

Usage:

1. Combine ingredients. Add 1- 2 teaspoons to bath1 teaspoon to a foot bath. It can also be used as massage oil or add 1 to 2 teaspoons to your bath. Patchouli is optional on account of its overwhelming smell so do not use if you cannot stand it.

Essential Oil Preparation For Painful Periods/Cramps

Clary Sage/Cypress: 2-4 drops

Usage:

Apply topically to the abdomen. Next, use a warm compress on the abdomen.

Varicose Veins Essential Oil Blend

Veins in the body may become weakened with time and lots of pressure. As a result, they become enlarged and twisted.

Cypress essential oil - 30 drops,

Lavender - 20 drops

Lemon essential oil- 10 drops

Coconut oil - 2 oz

Usage:

1. Blend all and apply morning and night. Improvement will be noticeable in about a month.

2. When this happens, apply daily for 3 or 4 months more.

Candida Or Yeast Infection
Lemon essential oil - 5 drops

Melaleuca essential oil - 5 drops

Oregano essential oil - 3 drops

Usage:

1. Add the essential oils to a gel cap then take internally two times daily for about 10 to 14 days.

2. Take a two weeks break then repeat the procedure.

Vaginal Candida Or Yeast Infection Douche
Geranium essential oil - 1 drops

Tea Tree essential oil - 2 drops

Rosemary essential oil - 2 drops

Lavender essential oil - 2 drops

Vinegar - 2 tablespoons

Lukewarm water - 3 cups

Usage:

1. Mix ingredients together.

2. Use once daily as a douche or Sitz bath.